OBESE TO THIN BODY

IN

90 DAYS

1

OBESE TO THIN BODY

IN

90 DAYS

BY

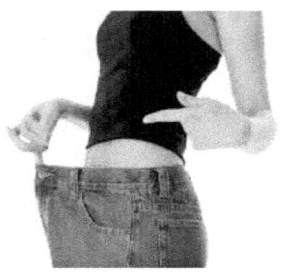

DAVID A. OSEI

OBESE TO THIN BODY *IN* 90 DAYS

Effective roadmap to fastest weight-loss unto perfect body

Copyright 2015 by David A. Osei

Twitter: @davidakufoo

All materials in this book are non-fiction and are primarily based on practical personal cycling experience, applying road safety regulations and others' life experiences on London urban roads.

First published on Kindle, Amazon.com

Contact Author: Name: David A. Osei , Email: davidoseia@gmail.com

<u>Dedication</u>

I dedicate this book **'OBESE TO PERFECT BODY** *IN* 90 DAYS' to all big gals who unfortunately have lost their dear lives, all present obese and to all potential obese in the nearest future. You must live and not die. Your health is my grave concern.

Thank You!!

Table of Contents

Preface

This book is based practically on helping obese people in the world to also achieve perfect (thin) body desirable to all eyes and people. Clinically, you are declared obese when your body weight is over 20% higher than normal body weight. Obesity kills people and also subjects many to countless of diseases such as blood pressure, diabetic and stroke to mention a few. All these problems are causing lives worth living dying needlessly.

Majority of obese people have tried and tested several suggestions, supplements, dietary patterns and fortunes with the desire to lose weight but sometimes leave them with fast deteriorating health and hopelessness. I honestly want to assure you that by following the steps in this book, you will achieve your dream of perfect health, body, weight-loss and strength needed for long life.

'Knowledge is power only when it is applied accordingly'. Knowing is not doing, but doing after knowing. Healthy lifestyle is paramount, hence read this book and apply the knowledge accordingly with determination. Let's make obesity zero death. Thanks!!

The Benefits of This Book

Exceptionally, these are the various benefits to be derived from reading this book:

- Firstly, this book unveils the causes of obesity.
- Secondly, it throws light on the health disastrous effect of obesity.
- Thirdly, it reveals the plan for tackling obesity in your body.
- Apart from this, the book teaches on how to effectively lose weight in 90 days and achieve thin body.
- Also, how to maintain the attained thin body.
- Ultimately, the benefits of attaining perfect body.

Why This Book?

This book is written to help obese people rediscover confidence and hope of new better chapter in their lives. It is aimed at bringing to light other possible workable alternative to losing weight fast. I personally use this plan and honestly, it has been significantly helpful to me. I believe by following the detailed weight-loss plan and steps in this book, it will go a long way to rid yourself of unwanted pounds that you carry along all the time. **Many thanks for downloading this book. Thanks!!**

Chapter 1

What Is Obesity?

An obese person is somebody who has accumulated so much body fat that it might have a negative effect on their health. If a person's bodyweight is at least 20% higher than it should be, he or she is considered obese. If your Body Mass Index (BMI) is between 25 and 29.9 you are considered overweight.

If your BMI is 30 or over you are considered obese. Clinical research and practice demands that individual body weight should range between certain acceptable level. By weighing beyond the BMX, you are clinically obese. Weight gain is caused by so many factors. Below are some of them:

Causes of Obesity

Genetics

Obesity has a strong genetic component. Offsprings of obese parents are much more likely to become obese than offsprings of lean parents.

This is not to say that obesity is completely predetermined because our genes aren't as set in stone as you may think. The signals we send our genes can have a major effect on which genes are expressed and which are not.

Consuming too many calories

Eating too much because of uncontrollable appetite for food can lead to obesity. As you eat more food, you indirectly consume more calories and that brings about obesity. This used to be the case just in developed nations - however, the trend has spread worldwide. Being gluttonous is not helpful to one's health.

Eating Too Much Junk Food

Today, foods are often little more than refined ingredients mixed in with a bunch of chemicals. These products are engineered to be cheap, last long on the shelf and taste so incredibly good that we just can't get enough. Junk foods are always saturated with fatty stuff that eventually builds up in the body.

Trauma

Distressing events-such as childhood sexual, physical, or emotional abuse; loss of a parent during childhood; or marital or family problems-can contributes to overeating and eventually obesity.

Alcohol

Alcoholic beverages such as: beer, wine, and mixed drinks are very high in calories.

Medicines or medical conditions

Some medical conditions and medicines may also cause weight gain. Examples include having Cushing's syndrome or hypothyroidism or taking certain antidepressants or corticosteroids.

Not sleeping enough

If you do not sleep enough your risk of becoming obese doubles, according to research carried out at Warwick Medical School at the University of Warwick. Professor Francesco Cappuccio evidence clearly showed that sleep deprivation significantly increase obesity risk in both children and adults.

Your friends and family

If they eat a lot of snack foods high in saturated fat, eat at irregular times, and skip meals, you probably will too. And if they are not physically active, you may not be either.

Low self-esteem

Being overweight or obese may lower your self-esteem and lead to eating as a way to comfort yourself. Repeated failure at dieting also can affect your self-esteem and make it even harder to lose weight.

Emotional concerns

Emotional stress, anxiety, or illnesses such as depression or chronic pain can lead to overeating. Some people eat to calm themselves, to avoid dealing with unpleasant tasks or situations, or to dampen negative emotions.

Trauma

Distressing events—such as childhood sexual, physical, or emotional abuse; loss of a parent during childhood; or marital or family problems—can contribute to overeating.

Smoking

Some people gain weight when they stop smoking. One reason is that food often tastes and smells better after quitting smoking.

Another reason is because nicotine raises the rate at which your body burns calories, so you burn fewer calories when you stop smoking. However, smoking is a serious health risk, and quitting is more important than possible weight gain.

Age

As you get older, you tend to lose muscle, especially if you're less active. Muscle loss can slow down the rate at which your body burns calories. If you don't reduce your calorie intake as you get older, you may gain weight.

Midlife weight gain in women is mainly due to aging and lifestyle, but menopause also plays a role. Many women gain about 5 pounds during menopause and have more fat around the waist than they did before.

Pregnancy

During pregnancy, women gain weight to support their babies' growth and development. After giving birth, some women find it hard to lose the weight. This may lead to overweight or obesity, especially after a few pregnancies.

Sporting Activity

Certain sporting activity demands the athletes put on certain magnitude of weight in order to be competitive. Some of the sports are: Wrestling, Judo, Weightlifters, to mention a few.

The above mentioned are some of the causes of obesity that can affect anybody if care is not exercised. Below underline some of the effects obesity brings to its sufferers.

Effects of Obesity

The effects of obesity are enormous and extremely detrimental to the health of sufferers. When one is clinically declared obese, the following effects are likely to impact on the person's health, even though not only these:

- High blood pressure
- Diabetes (type 2 diabetes)
- Heart diseases (Atherosclerosis– heart attack)
- Joint problems (osteoarthritis)
- Sleep apnea (breathing interruptions)
- Cancer (breast, colon and prostate cancers)
- Metabolic syndrome (cardiovascular disease)
- Psychosocial effects
- Stroke

- High total cholesterol

The above are some of the health detriments from obesity. The next chapters would detail the plan of execution needed to rid oneself of obesity within 90 days. However, even though the plan is effective and workable, there are several obstacles that obese people have to overcome to achieve their perfect body. Below are some in extreme cases:

Chapter 2

Obstacles To Perfect Body

This book is designed to help obese people overcome this unfortunate phenomenon plighting their lives. Apparently, this weight-loss concept designed in this book is efficient enough to treat obesity and eventually provide perfect body shape and health to practitioners. The major hindrances to this effective plan that can cause practitioners to either stop or never try at all are numerous.

Nevertheless, by overcoming these obstacles you are surely on course to losing weight and achieving your dream perfect body. Some factors to discourage implementation of this fat reduction concept are:

Laziness

Laziness is one of the discouraging factors that prevent people from sticking to this plan to lose weight and attain their dream body. That is getting up to stick to this plan is not easy. Everybody likes easy going life. Not having to do so much but achieve your goals. I like it and everybody does, so do your best to conquer laziness and go ahead with the plan.

Fear

Everybody, one way or the other has an element of fear that prevents him from doing something of wants. It is important not to yield to element of fear any time you desire to execute this plan.

Discouragement

It is possible to get discouraged in the course of this program especially when you are not immediately getting morale support and encouraging yourself. You would in this case need perseverance to get there.

Lack of funds

Another hindrance is lack of money to effectively carry out this plan. Not having money would definitely deter you from going ahead with this plan. You need money to acquire all the necessary items and equipments to perfectly execute this plan. Comparatively, you do not need huge sums of money to participate in this program.

Lack of Practical Experience

It is important to know how to carry out this plan. Any way it is not difficult to get started and learn how to practically do it. You can get discouraged if you are not determined to learn how to execute it without first knowing how. Nevertheless, there is useful alternative.

Not surrendering comfort zone

Very often, it is not all that easy to surrender your comfort zone to take up another trend. Even though this is clearly a problem, it is possible to overcome it and start something new that would impact positively on your life. Come out of your comfort zone and make it work.

Family commitments

Especially, if unfortunately you are so much involved in caring for your little kids, time would be a serious problem since you must always be with them. However, the alternative can be the solution. That is not being outdoors but indoors to execute this plan for perfect body.

Peer pressure from friends

Evidently, if you are the type who is in the group of friends with similar obese problem, peer pressure can derail this program. A lot of people do listen, watch and follow what friends do and so can be derailed especially if encouragement is not given by these trusted friends. Be concerned about your perfect body and health not others. On the other hand, if you are lucky to receive support that would be great. Even if none is given go ahead and pursue your healthy lifestyle dream.

Not sticking to the Plan of action

Another possible obstacle is not being dedicated to the outlined plan of execution. For rapid results it is recommended to stick to the detailed plan of action. Alternatively, you can stick to your own reformed plan but probably that would delay the desired results especially not being consistent and serious.

It is important that you do not allow the above mentioned obstacles to hinder your desire to lose weight and live a healthy life with perfect body frame.

The next chapter describes in detail the plan of action to achieve your perfect body frame.

Chapter 3

The Plan Of Action

This plan of action is what I myself use to always control my body weight not to become overweight and obese. It has been very effective for me without having to spend fortune on dietary supplements which eventually do not work. This efficient weight control and loss plan would last 90 days within which you would immediately see unprecedented results compared to other weight-loss plans.

My effective plan for the unprecedented attainment of weight-loss is **cycling-to-sweat** for a period of 90 days continuously. Cycling is not a thing for some people and at a mention of it many people just dislike it. I must be honest with everybody that it is one of the fastest means to shed off unnecessary body weight. The primary goal is to generate heat in the body to fight the body fat residue.

As you cycle around, your system generates heat and so affects any organ in the body not exempting fat residues. The fat element usually builds up on the internal body organs sometimes inhibiting its efficient functioning. In every human body frame, it contains some level of fat to cushion the outer layer. However, the excess fat is what makes the body to balloon to obesity weight.

The reason why this plan works successfully is that, we all understand that obesity is derived from excessive fat which is the residue of saturated oil, animal fat, fatty foods and other fats elements that pile up in the body and continue to expand the outer layers of the body. Fat is a soluble element. This saturated fat melts away any time something hot affects it. Comparatively, just like normal butter melting as a result of heat from fire or scorching sun.

This is similar to the piled up fat in the body. Cycling is a form of exercise that generates heat in the body. As the body generates continuous heat, all these hidden piled up stubborn fat begins to gradually melt away. That is why people who cycle a lot mostly look fit and strong by virtue of constant burning off fat in their body enabling the body system to function properly.

Getting Started

To effectively get started and execute this plan, first and foremost, you ought to acquire a bicycle of any kind, Road bike or mountain bike to mention a few. In addition to bicycle are helmet, high-vis/reflectors, pollution mask, cycling goggles, bottle of water, bicycle puncture kits, body weight gauge and attire.

With respect to executing this plan domestically, the items you would need are: domestic standing bicycle to be fixed at home, bottle of water, towel, cycling shoe and body weight gauge. Because it is at home, casual attire is recommended except you desire special one. Actually, there are no need for other things like helmet, high-vis/reflectors, puncture kits and others since you are not stepping out.

REQUIRED ITEMS

1   2   3

4   5   6

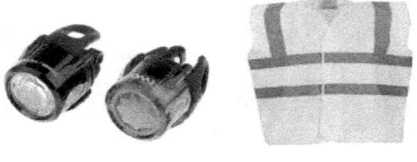 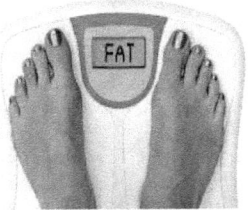

7   8   9

1. Road Bicycle   2. Standing Bicycle

   3. Bicycle Goggle   4 Bicycle Helmet

   5. Bicycle Water Bottle   6. Pollution Mask

   7. Bicycle Lights   8. Hi-Vis/Reflect

   9. Weight Gauge

These are the only things needed for the start of this plan. After acquiring these things respectively, you then have to follow any of the underscored cycling plans to achieve the perfect body goal.

Now, therefore, the respective cycling plans to follow are:

Plan A – Cycle To Work

Firstly, the Plan A in this perfect body program is to cycle to work. Do your best to stop driving, motorcycling and taking public transport to work especially if the distance is not too far away. If your workplace distance is up to 14 miles, that would be tremendously effective. At this distance, the body temperature would shoot up and generate extensive heat to start burning off the stubborn fat deposits in the body by melting them away.

However, if cycling on main road is not your thing, not confident and brave enough, too old to be on the road from all indications as well as being incapable to ride as a consequence of the farther distance, there are other alternative cycling plans of execution. Read on.

Plan B – Cycle at Community parks

Secondly, another place you can comfortably cycle is community parks. In fact if you feel riding on the roads are not safe for you and that you do not have the confidence to do so, use community parks as alternative convenient places to cycle to achieve your perfect body. This can be done in the mornings, afternoons, evenings and over the weekend depending on your time schedule if cannot cycle every day to work. It apparently serves the same purpose when appropriately done.

Plan C – Cycle on Greenways Route

Thirdly, in Britain there are thorough designed Greenways route that run through boroughs to the city that cyclists and individuals use to travel to the city and other places in London if they do not want to use the main roads. At these routes, cycling does not get interrupted by cars or any other major road users. Cycling there is safe and convenient apart from parks. All that you do is cycling from one end to another or preferred distances. I do it sometimes. It is safe.

Plan D – Cycle within Neighborhood Streets

Also, other places cycling can take place are quiet Neighborhood streets that are not much busy with cars so that the plan execution is not extremely interfered.

Plan E – Cycle at Hilly terrain

Apart from this, riding safely at hilly terrain is another effective technique to achieve the perfect body. Cycling at hilly terrain accelerates generation of heat which burns off the stubborn fat residue in the body as a result of excessive exertion of power and energy during climbing.

Plan F - Cycle on bush paths/roads

Besides this, cycling on bush paths and roads can be beneficial if any of the above mentioned places are not convenient or cannot be accessed. Bush roads and paths are sometimes quiet and devoid of tremendous interferences and disturbances from other road users.

Plan G – Cycle at Home

Another convenient place this effective cycling plan can be carried out is your own home. If outdoor cycling is not your thing, acquire standing bicycle equipment to fulfill this plan and achieve your perfect body. This plan is helpful to excessive obese individuals who struggle to walk about and those who dislike outdoor cycling.

As you manage to mount on the standing bike, you can execute the plan comfortably in your own home without stepping out. It is also recommendable to all those who do not know how to cycle at all. Among all the above mentioned cycling techniques, cycling at home is most convenient and peaceful except distraction from family members.

Plan D – Join Cycling Club

In addition to the above, joining cycling club in your town or community can be equally helpful in a situation where you feel lazy to cycle around alone. I am talking about effective cycling club that cycle or race every weekend. It should be active cycling club.

Plan E – Cycle on Weekends

Also, if you cannot execute the plan by cycling-to-sweat during the week days, then put in much effort over the weekend to compensate for the lost time during the week days. In that case you have to cycle for long hours to generate the required amount of heat to burn off the fat deposit in the body.

How To Execute The Perfect Body Plan

The perfect body plan is to achieve a certain level of heat in the body to burn off the fat residue. Below are some of the ways to attain that:

Cycle to sweat

The first most important factor to consider in this perfect body exercise is cycling to sweat at any time. Cycling casually would not yield this vital requirement necessitated for this program. As you cycle till sweating point, you burn off the stubborn body fat accumulated in the body because of excessive heat generated.

Cycle at Speed

It is not just cycling around that does the trick. Even though not emphatically brushing off any kind of cycling, it is a pinpoint strategy to cycle at speed on a level terrain in order to actually generate heat and sweat which is parallel to hilly terrain. By casually cycling around without sweating, you can hardly generate the needed body heat to effectively burn off the fat residue in the body.

Cycle at long distance

Do your best to cycle at long distances. By cycling at long distance, you are likely to sweat profusely which is recommended for perfect body plan of execution.

Cycle at hilly terrain

Cycling at hilly terrain helps to generate heat and sweat fast and easily. Climbing hills at force demands exertion of pressure and that helps in this direction.

Cycle for long hours

If you are executing this plan at level terrain, cycle for hours in order to generate maximum heat in the body. Unlike hilly terrain where you have to use extra energy which quickly generates enough heat to attack the body fat, cycling long hours can be of help to attain that.

Drink lots of water

As you continue to cycle for long hours and sweating alongside, drink more water in order to sweat more.

Eating Habit During Plan of Action

Cut down fatty foods: It is advisable to cut down fatty foods during this plan of execution. I am not expressly declaring halt to eating your favorite fatty foods. But I mean reduce the quantity for the time being during this program.

Eat mostly fruits and vegetables: I am not suggesting stop eating your favorite fatty foods altogether, however, for the sake of this program eat more fruits and vegetables to compensate for the fatty foods you have reduced.

Drink more water: Drink more water and urinate more. This helps to free the body of any unwanted elements in the body.

Chapter 4

The Plan, Activities and Results

Below outlines the detailed plan of execution and the results likely to achieve if the plan is strictly adhered to:

Week	Hours	Activity	Results
1	5 – 10	Cycle to Sweat	Reduction of fat
2	5 – 10	Cycle to Sweat	Reduction of fat
3	5 – 10	Cycle to Sweat	Reduction of fat
4	5 – 10	Cycle to Sweat	Reduction of fat
5	5 – 10	Cycle to Sweat	Reduction of fat
6	5 – 10	Cycle to Sweat	Reduction of fat
7	5 – 10	Cycle to Sweat	Reduction of fat
8	5 – 10	Cycle to Sweat	Reduction of fat
9	5 – 10	Cycle to Sweat	Reduction of fat
10	5 – 10	Cycle to Sweat	Reduction of fat
11	5 – 10	Cycle to Sweat	Reduction of fat
12	5 – 10	Cycle to Sweat	Reduction of fat
13	Total hours= 60 -120		Perfect body attained

In the course of executing this plan, if you reach the level of your wanted body perfection you can stop it even before the 90 days limit. In the event of experiencing complications during execution of this plan, stop and consult your doctor.

Importantly, the success of this plan depends largely on how you stick to the plan of execution and efficient way of implementing it. It is possible not to reach your body perfection at 90 days depending on execution pattern by you, but continue the process and assuredly you would reap the desired results.

Month By Month Results

By sticking to this pattern of action, week by week, month by month it is expected that there would be continuous tremendous change in the body shape.

Evidently, in the first week your body would start experiencing some pains and discomfort. This is normal because of the constant cycling pushing the body to unknown territory. If you begin to feel bodily pains, take some pain killers to relieve the body of excessive pain. During the pain period, do not abandon the plan of action, however, be determined, persist and persevere. Some parts of the body that you would feel pains are: the thighs, bum, the hands as well as the entire body.

In the second week, the body would gradually be adjusting to the strenuous pressure it has been subjected into. The pain would subside and everything becoming normal. At this point, the body would have adjusted and fat burning process already taken place making the plan of action not a tedious activity anymore.

Of the first month, not only would you see significant fat deposit in the body shrinking, your fitness level would improve as well as your health. In the first month, it is expected that the fat residue would shrink by 30 percent depending on the extent to which you aggressively follow the above plan of action. Prior to starting this program, weigh yourself to determine the body fat index to enable you monitor the steady reduction of it weekly.

In the second month at which time you are well above the halfway of the plan of action, the fat deposit would have shrunk massively revealing all the body hidden curves you crave for. At this point, your fitness would continue to improve including your health. The excess body weight is expected to have shrunk by 50 to 70 percent on course to the level of perfect body you desire.

Ultimately, at the end of the third month, it is expected that the body built-up fat would have reduced shrinking the entire body weight including both the abdomen and the stomach. Consequently, this would reveal the hidden natural body curves dislodged by the obesity. At this stage it is estimated that the excess body weight would have shrunk by 90 to 100 percent or 20 pounds. This should be enough to give you the perfect body you crave for. That is thin body with curves, looking young, beautiful, muscular and robust.

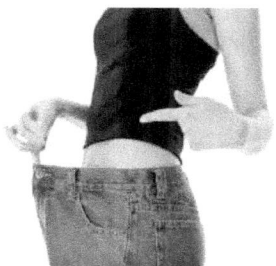

The Perfect Body Outlook

The perfect body concept is the level at which your body weight index shrinks to personally acceptable level. When the body fat shrinking process reaches pleasant and comfortable level, you can scale back the plan of action and live a normal life. After achieving the desired perfect body frame, the following underscored becomes undeniable results:

- The fat level in the body reduces to at least 90 percent making it less fatty.
- The body curves appear exposing all the hidden body gems you naturally possess.
- The body fitness improves and becomes robust.
- The immune system is strengthened to fight any ailment that encroaches on the body system.
- All already existing ailments in the body starts disappearing making way for better health.
- The body becomes beautiful, muscular and looking younger than its age. It delays in ageing giving you time to enjoy beauty and pleasantries.
- Ultimately, the general health of the body is always perfect and above board in its index comparison.

These are the benefits that perfect body offers to anybody who desires it. The above proposed plan of action has the capacity to produce all these body perfection results.

Maintaining Your Body Perfection

Maintaining your body perfection frame after diligently attaining it is one of the most important facets of this program. After arduous attainment and carelessly letting all your efforts go in vain within months triggering demand for fresh start all over again is totally undeserved, hence, to maintain your body perfection frame, follow these steps:

Cut down eating fatty foods: Do your best to cut down the fatty foods. I certainly do not imply stop your favorite foods. Eat, but not too much fatty foods.

Cut down eating fatty meat: Fatty meat should be reduced drastically. Eating fish, chicken and less fatty meat is better than red fatty meat.

Continue the plan of execution: That is, continue the **cycle-to-sweat** regime occasionally. You can reduce the number of hours from five to ten hours to three to six hours weekly.

Eat more vegetables and fruits: Eat more vegetables and fruits to compensate for the fatty foods stopped.

Cut down sugar and salt levels: Eat less sugar and salt.

The Benefits of Cycle-To-Sweat

There are numerous benefits to derive from Cycle-to-sweat plan of execution and below are some:

Losing weight

The primary goal of this concept is to lose weight. The first and foremost benefit of this concept is weight-loss and gaining perfect body. As the body continues to shrink of its fat deposit, the body system begins to lose weight leading to perfect body frame.

Saves money

This plan would save you fortune which would have been used to buy dietary supplements which eventually never works. They in reality do not burn off any fat in practice, but this plan does successfully. Also you do not need gym membership to accomplish this plan which charges for membership.

Improving Fitness

After significant reduction of fat deposit in the body, it paves way for good healthy lifestyle. When the body organs inwardly become free from fatty elements, they are able to function efficiently improving the fitness of the body. This makes the body frame as fit as fiddle at all times.

Not vulnerable to common disease

As your health and fitness improve, it builds the body immune system making it resistant to common diseases. This helps to prevent constant medication which is not conducive for the body considering the side effects thereof.

Long life

By keeping fit and healthy, it becomes a recipe for long life. You are likely to live longer than unhealthy looking person who is obese.

Improving general health

This plan has the potential to improve the general body system. That is, as the fat deposit level gradually decreases, the various organs in the body frame begin to have the freedom to function properly. The lever operates well, the blood circulation flows smoothly, the veins become non-clotted, diabetes and high blood pressure disappear, kidney and joint problems get controlled.

Improves Sexual life

Sexual underperformance is one of the major problems that face many people in relationship. Excessive body fat deposit can be one of the causes of sexual underperformance. By implementing this plan to shed off the body fat residue, the sexual connecting organs become free and active potentially resulting in improved sexual performances.

Real Life Changing Story

This real life story is about a friend of mine who was also obese. He constantly saw me cycling almost every time to work. He kept enquiring about the distance I do cover to work on my bike and other places I visit in London, UK. I told him everything about cycling, the importance of it and how it helps me in so many ways.

Little did I know that his unrelenting questioning was a recipe for extracting in depth information about the benefits of cycling. Within no time, he had stopped using public transport to work and started cycling. To my utter surprise, within a month to two, I vividly saw a massive change in his body.

He had shed off much excess weight and reduced in stature. His body looked muscular and in perfect shape, fit and healthy entirely different from the previous times. I was not so much surprised because I had been experiencing that myself. This is not an exaggeration but a fact. I want to encourage you to take the pain and stick to the pattern of the weight-loss plan outlined above and see whether you would not have a life changing story to share with friends and families

The next chapters provide guidance on **how to cycle safely on road** so that your plan of execution can be implemented safely without any problem.

Chapter 5

Before Implementation

Checking the Condition of the Bicycle

Prior to setting off on your bike to begin this plan of action, there is the need to check the condition of the bike so that it does not fail in the course of this important plan.

- First and foremost, ensure that the brakes on the bike are working perfectly.
- Check also the bicycle front and rear lights. In case they are not brightening properly, change the battery so that they do so.
- Apart from this, examine the neck of the bike if it is loose so that it can be tightened.
- In addition, check both the back and front hub if they are also loose.
- Ensure that the tyres both front and back are well inflated and that they are free from punctures.
- Check the bolts tightening both the back and front wheels.
- Be sure the bell is working fine.
- Is the chain well oiled? Dry chains are not good for comfortable cycling.
- Both the pedal and the crank need to be checked in case the bolts holding them tight are coming loose.
- Is the seat bolt well tightened in position?

Embarking on this thorough bike examination is not time wasting but good for safety riding. It would be very disappointing having started the execution and you end up having to abandon it as a consequence of bicycle performance failure.

Things you should have before Setting off

Prior to setting off, it is recommended to have the following bicycle kits on you:

- Puncture Kits/Basic tools.
- Bicycle Pump if you are to cycle afar.

- Bottle of Water.
- Wear both your helmet and the Hi-vis vest/ reflectors .
- Bicycle lock if at some point you have to lock it outside.
- And public transport pass if you are going afar in case the bicycle breaks down and you cannot fix it immediately and continue.

These above mentioned items are helpful in cycling. After having all these stuff with you, it is time to set off to the implementation of the plan.

Chapter 6

Time of Implementation

Qualities of a Cyclist

To effectively execute the plan, it is desirable to possess the following qualities when cycling:

- Be courageous
- Be positive
- Be patient
- Be sensible
- Be confident
- Be instinctive
- Be willing to learn
- Be safety minded
- Be obedient
- Be sharp and reactive
- Be alert and focus

These various qualities would facilitate and promote fullest concentration and focus on the road. It would be advisable not to underestimate the above mentioned qualities.

Now on the Road

When you start executing this plan by being on the road with your bicycle, do your best to consider the following careful for the sake of safety.

- Stay in the bicycle lanes, route and tracks.
- In the event that there are no earmarked cycle lanes whilst on the road, do your best to stay close to the kerp or yellow lines.
- Avoid car lanes and stay in the bus lanes.

- Obey all road traffic regulations without ignoring any of them.
- Do your best not to jump red lights. It is a dangerous thing to do.
- Occasionally, check your back for traffic from behind.
- When approaching road junctions and intersections, it is advisable to slow down and check for cars coming from the junction roads.
- Alternatively, check your back and see if there are speeding cars in the car lane. If there are none, enter the car lane and keep away from the junction, but return to the cycle lane after safely passing the junction.
- In a situation where you have to cross outer car lanes to the other, check your shoulders and be sure there are no cars close by in both the outer car lanes and the car lane you are crossing to. Sufficiently give signals till the cars behind pick it up and slow down for you to cross safely. Don't just enter the car lanes without first checking for safety.
- Alternatively, wait till it is safe for you to cross without problems.
- If it happens that you are not confident enough to do so, dismount and use pedestrian zebra crossing to cross to the other side of the road.

Riding round Roundabouts

Sometimes riding round roundabouts can be extremely tricky. Unfortunately, accidents involving cyclist do occur at such places. So do go round roundabouts with extra caution in order to avoid accidents. To do so safely, stick to these steps:

- In the event that there is layout cycle lane, go round the roundabout using the cycle lanes.
- If there is no cycle lane, stay close to the kerb or the yellow lines to go round it.
- However, if you are to use car outer lane, stay in the middle of the outer lane behind cars till you exit the roundabout.
- Alternatively, use the outer car lane by giving signal to cars behind your course of direction.
- After going round the roundabout, exit and safely stay in the bicycle lane or close to the kerb to continue the journey.

Chapter 7

The Plan In Different Conditions

Cycling During Rainy Time

This concept can be implemented at any time. Below outlines some useful tips to cycle in rainy time:

- Slowing down to controllable speed is desirable. Depending on individuals, ride at a speed that you can comfortable manage without accident.
- Brake from afar and gently before hard braking in order to avert sliding because of the slippery surface of the road.
- Extra care should be exercised when doing overtaking. Unnecessary and unsafe overtaking is not advised.
- Switch on your rear light so that you can be seen
- Wear Hi-Vis/Reflectors
- Wear Rain Coat to prevent getting soaked wet
- Wear Cycle Goggles to prevent dirt entering into your eyes if necessary.
- Wear cycle pollution mask to prevent dirt entering your nozzle whilst breathing.

Cycling In Foggy Weather

To cycle in foggy weather condition safely, the following tips can also be helpful:

- Turn on both the front and rear bicycle lights because of poor visibility.
- Wear Reflector/Hi-Vis so that you can be seen by other approaching road users like cars, motorcycles and Lorries.
- Speed at a controllable speed that you are comfortable with.
- It is advisable that the bicycle brakes are efficient so that you can brake effectively.
- Wear Helmet as usual.

Cycling During Winter Condition

It is very tricky to cycle during winter condition but it is still possible to do so. To cycle safely in winter, apply some of these steps:

- In the same way, cycle at a controllable and comfortable speed so that you can safely handle emergencies.
- If it has snowed, ride at the gritted parts and not the snowy parts of the road.
- Avoid the Icy parts altogether, but if for some reason you have to ride there, exercise extra care so that you do not slide and fall off.
- It is advisable to start braking from afar and gently in order to avert sliding and fall offs.
- Wear Hi-Vis so that you can be seen.
- Turn on both the front and rear bicycle lights in order that you can be seen.
- Wear thick protective cloth to keep the body warm, wear hand gloves and warm shoes.

Cycling in Windy Conditions

Cycling in windy condition is no different from other treacherous conditions already mentioned. Some useful tips to consider are as follows:

- It becomes so difficult riding when you are unfortunately facing the wind direction.
- Riding becomes very easy and enjoyable when not facing the wind. In that case the wind pushes you and speeding become easy. Every cyclist loves it including myself.
- When the wind direction is from the side, you have to hold the steering firmly so that the bicycle direction is not controlled by the wind. The worse of it is that you can fall off.
- The brakes ought to be efficient in order to control any level of uncertainties.
- If the windy condition becomes unbearable and dangerous, find a safe place to hide till condition becomes normal and make cycling possible.
- Don't forget to wear your hi-vis/reflectors so that you can be seen in distance.
- Advisably, wear cycle pollution mask in order to avert dirt blowing into your nozzle or become part of your breathing.
- Wear Cycle Goggles to avert dirt entering your eyes to blur your vision on the road if any, not compulsory though.

Chapter 8

Do It Yourself (DIY)

Causes of Constant Inner Tube Punctures

In the course of executing this plan, it would be disappointing and devastating if it is obstructed by flat tyre. For this reason, knowing the basic causes of punctures and avoiding them would be extra helpful to this plan. Some of the basic causes of punctures to consider are as follows:

- Tyres being so old and worn out as well as inner tubes.
- Running over sharp objects such as broken glasses, nails, needles, sharp gravels and stones.
- Running into potholes
- Protruding spokes piercing the inner tube
- Broken tyre ring piercing the inner tube.
- Colliding with hard objects

Puncture Prevention

In order to prevent constant punctures, the suggestions below could be enormously helpful.

- Use if possible tyre liners. You can use self-created tyre liner with your old tyres and tubes. Alternatively, use new original liners for your tires
- Avoid running over sharp objects and potholes.
- Use new tyres and inner tubes in case they are too old.
- Cut off all protruding spokes and put liner over it.

How to Fix a Punctured Inner Tube - DIY

a. Turn the bicycle upside down

b. Bring out your puncture kits
c. Remove one side of the tyre
d. Bring the inner tube out
e. Pump the inner tube hard to locate the punctured hole
f. Pour water on the inner tube to locate the puncture place
g. After locating the puncture, mark the place
h. Dry the puncture place and use sand paper to rough the place
i. Pour the glue moisture on the rough place and leave it to dry
j. After it dries, remove the patch protector and place it at the glued punctured hole place.
k. Press it hard to stick dry to the punctured place.
l. Leave it for a little while and that is it. Finished.
m. Put the tube and the tyre open side back in.
n. Pump the tyre and turn the bike up again, mount on it and off you go.

Treatment of the Chain

A bicycle chain is a roller chain that transfers power from the pedals to the drive-wheel of a bicycle, thus propelling it. To make the bike pedaling easy and comfortable without putting so much strain on the cyclist's legs, occasionally oil the chain.

Oiling the Chain

To ensure comfortable cycling whilst executing this plan is to occasionally oil the bicycle chain for smooth ride. This would prolong the health and life of the chain. As soon as you start experiencing hard pedaling and talking chain, oil the chain. To oil the chain, pour the bicycle chain oil on the chain slowly whilst turning the crank. If you use pressurized chain oil, press and keep turning the crank.

If you are using pouring chain oil, pour some of the oil into a small cup, use a toothbrush or brush to dip into it and rub it over the chain whilst turning the crank slowly. Do not turn the crank too fast otherwise the oil would come off and dry quickly.

Chapter 9

Your Directions

Ways To Give Signals

Is the process of telling other road users like cars, motorcyclists and many more your intending direction to go. Below are some **ways** to give signals:

- Use outstretched hand either right or left hand as the situation would require.
- It is possible to use either left or right leg to give direction but it is very uncommon.
- In addition, you can use your head to give valid signal to other road users by catching their eyes.
- It is advisable to check your shoulders first for safety from behind before acting upon it.

Vehicle Signals

- Vehicles also give signals to cyclists and other road users. Some commonest ones are:
- Left Indicator light means the driver is intending to go left
- Right indicator light means the driver is intending to go right
- Double indicator lights means stationary and caution.
- Flashing head lights means giving way to the other road user
- The double occasional red light means braking.
- Flashing siren light cars are emergency vehicles, such as Police, Fire Brigade, Ambulances and Doctors' cars to mention a few. They may be attending to emergency issues so give way.
- Lit double rear white lights means the car is reversing, so stay clear to avert collision.
- You can refer to the Highway Code book for more comprehensive vehicle signals and meanings.

Chapter 10

Knowing The Dangers

Apparently some of the common causes of cyclist's injuries and deaths are:

- Not obeying road traffic regulations can easily cause accidents and injuries and potentially deaths.
- Riding under the influence of stimulants such as: alcohol, banned drugs and anything that affects normal behavior.
- Straying into car lanes unexpectedly without first checking for safety.
- Staying in-between Lorries' blind side and the kerb. If the lorry moves without checking its mirror to give you enough space you can get crushed.
- Wrongly going round roundabouts. If you get it wrong and happen to collide with a car that would be seriously fatal.
- Another cause is crossing roads without first checking for safety first.
- Wrong road designs, signs and layouts, especially sections where they have been liberalized.
- Not constantly checking your shoulders before any maneuvers.
- Getting distracted on the road, depriving you of concentration and focus.
- Playing to the crowd as a hero can be fatal as well. Don't do it if it is not safe.
- Not wearing safety kits such as hi-vis, reflectors and helmet.
- No bicycle lights to alert your presence to oncoming road users.
- Lack of driving discipline from the drivers.
- Speeding at road intersections and junctions to beat red lights by drivers. Cars crossing cycle lanes on main roads junctions and crushing into it.

The above mentioned common causes of cyclists' deaths are few in the ocean so beware.

Going Through Cars (Beating Traffic)

In an event of heavy traffic on the way, it is possible to continue cycling by following these steps:

- If there are enough gaps between the cars, slowly ride through them.
- As soon as the cars start moving and the gap narrows, brake and stay behind cars till the gap opens again for you to go through them again.
- If one of the car lanes is less traffic and fast moving, filter through to join that and continue. Nonetheless, ensure that you ride in the middle of the lane behind cars instead of staying on the white dividing lines which would invariably allow cars to pass you by.
- Also, if there is cycle lane by the kerb and it is empty it should be used to continue, nevertheless, if it is occupy by a car, better use alternative means to continue.
- Another way of beating the traffic is, when the bicycle lane is occupied by a car, you can dismount, mount the pavement, push the bike pass the car occupying the cycle lane and then continue.
- After filtering through them, do your best to move to the bicycle lane or close to the kerb.

Racing Cars on the Road

Some drivers see it a great fun to race cyclist. It is not a good practice so when you find yourself in it, stay away from their lane and keep to your riding.

In most cases bus drivers do so. Whenever you see them passing you by and braking at bus stops at shorter distance in front of you, it is a clear sign the driver is racing you. Also, prevent you from passing them after stopping even though they have seen you clearly overtaking them they are racing you. Warn the drivers in their mirrors and either pull out of it or ask them to wait till you pass.

Dealing with Emergency Vehicles

Even though there could be no sounding siren, as soon as you spot emergency vehicles like Police, Ambulances, Fire Brigade and others, make sure you stay away from the middle of the road and let them pass just in case they are responding to emergencies. Do not obstruct them. Give them priority even if they intend you go first. Stop and let them go instead. Let them save a life dying.

Dealing with Lorries

Cycling round big Lorries can be tricky if not properly done. Some steps to follow are:

- Don't race Lorries. Be careful and avoid it altogether except they have stopped and it is safe to go round them.
- Don't stay in the kerb gap except there is an earmarked cycle lane and it is not occupied by a lorry.

- Stay behind them and wait if there is not enough gap for you to pass them by.
- Do check their indicator lights, so that you stay away from their intended direction.
- Avoid staying in the corners alongside them because if they should turn that direction you could be crushed.
- If Lorries intend to overtake you, stay out of their way and never enter into narrow gap with them.
- Give sufficient signal to them and make sure they have got the message before you act on it.

Chapter 11

General Implementation

At Traffic Lights

These are some guidelines as to how to cycle at traffic lights:

- Know where you are going since getting confused can be fatal
- Stay in front or behind cars which have stopped at the traffic lights
- Stay in the Outer Lanes to enable you move to the bicycle lane as soon as it is go.
- Check the cars' and vehicle's Indicator Lights so that you do not obstruct them if they are to turn the indicator's direction.

Doing Overtaking

Some useful tips to do overtaking are as follows:

- Ensure that it is safe first before doing the overtaking.
- Check vehicles' indicators so that you do not veered into their lane.
- Always check there is enough distance in front and back or on the side of the intended target before overtaking.

How to cycle on Pavement Cycle Lanes

There are some pavements which have both cycle lanes and pedestrian paths as well. To cycle on pavement bicycle lanes, follow these steps:

- Stay in the earmarked cycle lanes and leave the pedestrian paths for pedestrians.
- When you see pedestrians ahead, slow down to pass them.
- If you find pedestrians in the cycle lane, alert them of your presence using the bell.
- Use the pedestrian path in case the pedestrians are not leaving the cycle lane after alerting them.

- If pedestrians have spread across both cycle and pedestrian lanes, be patient and wait for them to give you way.
- When you come to a junction whilst on the pavement lane, look left and right before crossing it.
- If you find a car waiting to join the main road blocking your lane, cross the junction road from the cars' rear not the front.
- Alternatively, wait for the car to join the main road before you continue.

How to cycle round Parked and Moving Cars

To cycle safely around parked and moving cars, use the following steps:

- In the first place, check your back for safety before intending to ride round them.
- When passing by, do not be too close to them.
- Give enough space between you and the cars in case the driver opens the door unknowingly.
- Brake and wait behind parked cars if there is lorry passing by. This would give you enough room to cycle round the parked car.

Chapter 12

The Don'ts

Apparently, consider the following as no, no things to do whilst riding:

- Never take phone calls whilst riding.
- Avoid over speeding and cycle at controllable speed.
- Never ride on pavement without cycle lanes except possibly allowed.
- Never obstruct emergency cars. Give way to them.
- Never stay in the middle of the road to fix a bicycle problem. Find safer place to do so.
- Never ride in the dark without hi-vis, reflectors and bicycle lights on.
- Avoid rat racing vehicles. Keep away if you are being raced by them.
- Cross blocked junction cars from the rear not the front.
- Always stop and give priority to pedestrians when they are to cross or crossing the road.

References

1. Medical News Today (www.medicalnewstoday.com)
2. Stanford Healthcare.org (www.stanfordhealthcare.org)
3. National Heart, Lung and Blood Institute (www.nhlbi.nih.gov)
4. WebMD (www.webmd.com)
5. The Highway Code – United Kingdom
6. My Practical Cycling Experience On The Road

About The Author

The Author, David A. Osei is a keen weight control enthusiast who lives in London, United Kingdom. I love cycling to control my weight so that I don't become obese. It has been part of my pattern of weight control for years. Apart from this, I cherish sharing ideas and enormously assisting others to achieve their personal goals including healthy lifestyle.

With my vast cycling experience and knowledge about the impact it has on turning obese people's lives around, I deem it an immense responsibility to share my cycling knowledge and experience with obese people to enable them burn off body's stubborn fats deposit to promote healthy lifestyle and prevent untimely deaths anywhere in the world.

One Important Thing

Please having finished reading this book, I would be very grateful if you could spend some few minutes of your time and write a review for me.

This apparently would go a long way to enable me evaluate and ascertain the benefits and significant contribution my effort has made to readers like you.

I would highly appreciate your contribution and say thank you all the time for your help. Many thanks!!